Blue Zones

Lessons from the World's Longest-Living Communities

Sarah Wellness

Copyright © by **Sarah Wellness 2023.**

Disclosure Statement

Please be aware that the material in this publication is only intended for educational purposes. Every attempt has been made to offer accurate, current, trustworthy, and comprehensive information. Readers understand that the author is not giving out professional or medical advice. This book's information came from a variety of sources.

Table of Contents

Chapter 1: Blue Zones: Uncovering the Secrets of Exceptional Longevity

There are locations in the great tapestry of our planet where time appears to unfold at a different speed, where the rhythm of life pulses in tune with the soft pulse of longevity. These mysterious locations, dubbed "Blue Zones," have captured the attention of academics, scientists, and health enthusiasts alike.

We go on a voyage of discovery in this chapter, peeling back the layers of mystery that cloak these unique sites and setting the scene for a thorough inquiry into the teachings they contain for the search for a longer, healthier life.

They coined the phrase "Blue Zones" after embarking on a worldwide journey with a team of specialists to locate areas where people not only live longer but also flourish in amazing health and vigor. The name relates to the blue circles painted on maps to denote these remarkable locations, and it acts as a beacon urging us to discover their mysteries.

As we begin our journey, it is critical to grasp the parameters that characterize a Blue Zone. Buettner and his colleagues found particular places where individuals continuously live to be 100 years old or more, and do so with a quality of life that defies the typical aging trajectory. These people aren't just surviving; they're flourishing, with reduced incidence of chronic illnesses and better levels of well-being.

The chapter begins with a look at how the Blue Zones initiative came to be—a confluence of scientific investigation, cultural curiosity, and a common desire to discover the elixir of lasting health. We look at the project's origins, the careful research techniques used, and the tales of the people who kindled the interest that spurred the adventure to find the world's longevity hotspots.

The awareness that these Blue Zones are not the consequence of chance or luck is a recurring subject. Instead, they demonstrate the complex interaction of genetics, environment, lifestyle, and culture. We go into the nuances of this interaction, considering the elements that distinguish Blue Zones from the rest of the world, as well as the possible lessons they provide for transforming our own lives.

Furthermore, we investigate the Blue Zones concept's influence on public health, gerontology, and the larger scientific community. The discovery of these extraordinary societies has triggered a paradigm shift in our knowledge of aging and longevity, challenging conventional beliefs and sparking a communal desire for a deeper understanding of the human lifetime.

We build the framework for the next chapters in the spirit of this research, promising a full voyage through the Sardinian highlands, the Okinawa islands, the Californian enclave of Loma Linda, Costa Rica's Nicoya Peninsula, and the Greek refuge of Ikaria. Each of these Blue Zones has a unique tapestry of lessons to share, and our trip tries to unravel the threads that weave together to form the fabric of amazing longevity.

The mysteries of Blue Zones will be revealed as we progress through the chapters that follow, revealing not only the habits and practices that contribute to a long and vibrant life, but also the profound cultural and societal factors that highlight the importance of community, purpose, and connection in the pursuit of long-term well-being. The voyage into Blue Zones is a philosophical and cultural adventure that invites us to reconsider our attitude to health, aging, and the pursuit of a life well-lived.

Chapter 2: The Sardinian Secret: Nuoro, Italy - Discovering Centenarian Wisdom in the Heart of the Mediterranean

We find ourselves enveloped in the mystical embrace of Nuoro, a region that cradles the secrets of a unique community surviving far into their hundreds as we cross the sun-kissed hills and blue sky of Sardinia, Italy.

In this chapter, we go deep into the Sardinian Blue Zone, exploring the complexities of its culture, customs, and way of life that combine to create an unrivaled environment of longevity and well-being.

The Nuoro Landscape: Nature as a Fountain of Youth

Nuoro's rough topography and rolling landscapes serve as the backdrop for the narrative of Sardinian longevity. The clean, unpolluted air and the tranquility of the Mediterranean Sea provide a wonderful setting for a life of simplicity and peace with nature. We investigate the symbiotic interaction between the residents and their natural surroundings, pondering how a strong connection to the land adds to the people's lives.

The Centenarian Diet: Nourishment for the Soul and Longevity

The traditional food practiced by the Sardinian people is a cornerstone of the Sardinian secret.

We unravel the nutritional tapestry that preserves the vigor of Nuoro's centenarians by focusing on locally obtained, plant-based diets. We discover the culinary expertise that not only tantalizes the taste senses but also contributes to the remarkable health of the community, from the famed Cannonau wine, rich with antioxidants, to the richness of fresh vegetables and grains.

Nuoro's Social Tapestry of Community Bonds

Social links are more than just connections in Nuoro's close-knit communities; they are lifelines. We go deep into Sardinian villages, where extended families and strong friendships are the foundation of everyday life. The strong feeling of belonging and community spirit that pervades Nuoro contribute considerably to its citizens' general well-being.

We discover the social alchemy that turns simple existence into a vivid celebration of life via festivals, shared rituals, and a strong feeling of mutual support.

The Essence of Sardinian Longevity is Purposeful Living

In Nuoro, life is more than just a passing of time; it is a meaningful journey. We investigate the cultural fabric that connects work, family, and a strong sense of purpose, giving a road map for a meaningful and purpose-driven life.

The integration of everyday tasks with a feeling of responsibility and passion shows a holistic approach to life that goes beyond the commonplace, providing significant insights into the art of living well.

Rituals and Wisdom passed down through the generations

Nuoro is a live example of the preservation of time-honored customs. We unearth the traditions that have been treasured and handed down through generations, from storytelling to ancient dances. These rituals not only serve as a source of cultural identity, but they also play an important role in sustaining a feeling of continuity and connection to the past, which helps the Sardinian people's resilience and longevity.

As we near the end of our journey through Nuoro, we find ourselves immersed in a place where the air smells of centuries-old knowledge and the hills ring with the laughter of folks who have learned the art of aging gracefully.

Nuoro invites us to discover its secrets, to consider how a fusion of nature, nutrition, community, purpose, and tradition forms a timeless sanctuary where the goal of longevity is entwined with the very essence of life itself.

Chapter 3: Okinawa, Japan: The Immortal Island - Where Time Slows and Centuries Unfold

The fascinating archipelago of Okinawa sits on the far eastern horizon, where the Pacific Ocean caresses the beaches of Japan—an amazing sanctuary where time appears to flow at a different speed, and the search for immortality is not a simple ambition but a practical reality. We begin on an excursion into the heart of the Okinawa Blue Zone in this chapter, examining the cultural riches, lifestyle choices, and spiritual roots that have earned its residents the title **"The Island of Immortals."**

The Okinawan Seascape: A Tranquil Tapestry

The voyage into Okinawa starts with the turquoise expanse of the Pacific Ocean, which gently embraces this island paradise. Okinawa's seascape is more than just a geographical background; it is a living painting that sets the tone for its citizens' peaceful lives.

As we dive into Okinawans' connection with their marine environment, we discover the ocean's significant influence on their well-being and longevity, pondering the therapeutic harmony that comes from living in rhythm with the tides.

Ikigai: Okinawan Existence's Heartbeat

The notion of **"ikigai,"** a phrase that transcends linguistic barriers, and encapsulates the essence of finding pleasure, purpose, and satisfaction in daily life, is at the heart of Okinawan longevity. We investigate how ikigai is woven into Okinawa's cultural fabric, shaping the choices, vocations, and everyday activities of its residents. Okinawans not only add years to their lives but also life to their years, by pursuing meaningful undertakings and cultivating hobbies.

The Okinawan Diet: Longevity from the Earth and Sea

Okinawan cuisine develops as a gastronomic symphony that feeds both the body and the mind.

We tour Okinawa's colorful markets and family kitchens, learning the mysteries of their cuisine, with a concentration on nutrient-rich, plant-based foods. We dig into the nutritional treasure trove that forms the basis of Okinawan longevity, from the distinctive purple sweet potatoes to the enormous range of local vegetables and the omega-3-rich seafood derived from the surrounding waters.

Moai: Okinawan Resilience's Social Foundation

Okinawans practice the discipline of building **"moai"**—tight-knit social support groups that give companionship, emotional support, and a safety net throughout life's journey—in the sense of shared humanity. As we investigate the moai culture, we uncover how these intertwined webs of connections contribute to both mental and physical wellness.

The feeling of belonging and camaraderie that exists within these organizations attests to the value of social relationships in the quest for a long and active life.

Karate and Martial Arts: The Physical Immortality Dance

Martial arts are more than simply a physical exercise in Okinawa; they are a way of life. We go onto the dojo floors and training fields where generations have refined their bodies and souls via disciplines like Karate, reflecting on how these ancient practices contribute to Okinawan centenarians' resilience, flexibility, and strength. Physical activity combined with cultural heritage offers a comprehensive approach to well-being that goes well beyond the physical advantages of exercise.

Shisa and the Essence of Eternal Protection in Longevity Spirituality

We explore Okinawa's spiritual tapestry under the shadow of holy Shisa statues, a region where old beliefs and rituals coexist with the rhythms of contemporary life. Shisa, legendary animals said to fend off bad spirits, act as Okinawan dwellings' symbolic guardians. We unravel the threads linking the islanders to a deeper sense of purpose, calm, and the intangible aspects that contribute to their ageless existence as we dig into the spiritual rituals that pervade everyday life.

As we travel across Okinawa's lush landscapes, peaceful coasts, and old customs, the Island of Immortals invites us to consider not just the qualities that lead to longevity, but also the deep knowledge ingrained in its culture.

Okinawa, where time runs like a serene river, welcomes us to share its secrets, encouraging us to dance with the rhythms of life, grow our ikigai, and find the immortal essence that we all possess.

Chapter 4: Loma Linda, California: The Adventist Enclave - A Modern-Day Sanctuary for Longevity

A unique enclave arises in the heart of Southern California, buried inside the city of Loma Linda, where the golden colors of sunshine meet the mountainous landscape. This chapter tells the story of Loma Linda, a Blue Zone in the United States where the Seventh-day Adventist community has weaved a tapestry of longevity that defies contemporary life's speed.

As we begin our journey, the duality of history and development draws us in, exposing the secrets of a society that survives in the face of modern problems.

The Adventist Way of Life: A Plan for Health and Longevity

Loma Linda's Blue Zone status is inextricably linked to the lifestyle choices of its Seventh-day Adventist population. We dive into the key concepts of the Adventist lifestyle, in which a plant-based diet, frequent exercise, and a devotion to spiritual activities serve as daily cornerstones.

We discover the purposeful decisions that influence not just the physical health of Loma Linda inhabitants, but also their emotional and spiritual well-being as we explore the thriving farmers' markets and community events.

Rest, Renewal, and Longevity: The Sabbath Advantage

The Sabbath is central to the Adventist way of life—a day set apart for rest, meditation, and spiritual connection. We investigate the enormous influence of this deliberate stop on the community's overall health and lifespan. The Sabbath not only gives a respite from the strains of contemporary life, but it also develops a feeling of community and connectivity, which helps Loma Linda people cope with life's obstacles.

The Adventist Dietary Paradigm and Nutrition as Medicine

The chapter digs inside Loma Linda's kitchens and dining tables, revealing the nutritional concepts that drive the Adventist diet.

We uncover the dietary choices that have been associated with reduced incidence of chronic illnesses and greater life expectancy by focusing on plant-based foods, legumes, and fat moderation. The incorporation of nutrition as a type of preventative medicine, rather than merely subsistence, represents a paradigm change in how we understand the link between food and lifespan.

Faith as a Spiritual Anchor in a Modern World

In Loma Linda's spiritual core, we investigate the role of religion as a guiding factor in the lives of its citizens. The Seventh-day Adventist belief system impacts not just lifestyle choices but also mental resilience. It is based on a holistic perspective of health and well-being.

We explore how religion may serve as a spiritual anchor, offering strength and meaning as we negotiate the complexity of contemporary life via prayer, communal worship, and a common commitment to values.

A Modern Approach to Longevity Through Healthcare Innovation

Loma Linda's Blue Zone designation is due not just to healthy lifestyle choices, but also to the community's unique approach to healthcare. We visit cutting-edge medical institutions and research sites to see how advances in healthcare and dedication to preventative medicine contribute to the community's overall well-being.
In the face of current healthcare issues, the combination of modern medical research with holistic health practices demonstrates a forward-thinking approach to longevity.

Intergenerational Connections: Wisdom Passed Down Through the Generations

As we walk through Loma Linda's tree-lined lanes, we notice a feeling of continuity and intergenerational connection that defies the transience of contemporary life. Grandparents are involved in their grandchildren's lives, handing on not simply family customs but also a wealth of knowledge gained over decades of experience. We investigate the family relationships and feelings of heritage that pervade Loma Linda and contribute to the community's continuing vitality.

The Seventh-day Adventist community at Loma Linda, where tradition and modernity coexist, provides a model for modern-day longevity.

As we traverse the crossroads of religion, lifestyle, and healthcare innovation, the Loma Linda tale inspires us to reconsider our own choices and consider the possibility of peaceful coexistence of tradition and development with the goal of a longer, better life.

Chapter 5: Costa Rica's Nicoya Peninsula: The Peninsula of Life - Where Centenarian Wisdom Meets Pura Vida

The picturesque Nicoya Peninsula sits in the lap of the Pacific Ocean, where lush rainforests meet pristine beaches—a place where time dances to the beat of Pura Vida, where the pursuit of a long and vigorous life is not just a desire but an innate way of being.

This chapter immerses us in Nicoya's cultural richness, natural beauty, and centuries-old customs, revealing the secrets of a society that embodies the essence of longevity.

Pura Vida: Nicoya's Soulful Pulse of Existence

The vibrant rhythm of Pura Vida—a phrase that transcends its literal translation of "pure life" to encapsulate the Costa Rican philosophy of embracing life's simple joys, cultivating a positive outlook, and maintaining a laid-back, stress-free attitude— beats at the heart of Nicoya's longevity narrative. We start on a trip inside Nicoyans' everyday lives, where the spirit of Pura Vida intertwines with the fabric of life, leading to a holistic approach to well-being.

Centenarian Diets: Sabor Local Nourishing Body and Soul

The chapter develops as we go through Nicoya's busy marketplaces and traditional kitchens, discovering the gastronomic delicacies that are the region's staple diet.

We uncover the nutritional richness that supports Nicoyans, from the profusion of fresh fruits and vegetables to the traditional gallo pinto—a healthy combination of rice and beans. The focus on locally produced, whole foods is a celebration of the region's agricultural riches as well as a devotion to experiencing life's tastes.

Gardening in the Blue Zones: Getting Longevity from the Earth

Nicoyans' attachment to the land goes beyond the dinner table to the actual soil from when their food is derived. We dig into the Blue Zones gardening culture, in which people raise their fruits and vegetables, developing not just self-sufficiency but also a stronger connection to the natural environment.

Nicoyans have built a sustainable, agrarian lifestyle that not only feeds the body but also improves the soul via the knowledge handed down through generations.

Social Interaction: From Family to Community

Nicoya's life story is intertwined with strands of social connectedness that extend beyond family relationships to include the larger community. We discover the warmth of Nicoya's social fabric as we go through town squares and common areas. The links of family extend to neighbors, friends, and the larger community, forming a support network that promotes mental health, generates a feeling of belonging, and serves as a safety net for people at all stages of life.

Nature's Playground for Active Longevity: Outdoor Living

The chapter progresses as we discover Nicoya's rich surroundings, where nature is more than simply a background but a vital element of everyday life. Whether it's the joyful dance of traditional festivities or the energizing practice of traditional dance, Nicoyans enjoy outdoor activities that help them live active and healthy lives. The natural playground of Nicoya, with its golden beaches and lush rainforests, provides a canvas for a life lived in peace with nature.

Spirituality & Faith: Nicoya's Soul Sanctuary

The spiritual traditions that create a feeling of purpose, calm, and resilience contribute to Nicoya's Blue Zone designation. We dive into the religious traditions and beliefs that serve as the community's spiritual foundation. From exuberant fiestas to religious events, we investigate how religion serves as a source of strength, social connection, and a steadfast foundation in Nicoyans' life.

The Silver Age: Honoring Elders as Wisdom Pillars

Elders are venerated and cherished in Nicoya as the keepers of ancestral knowledge and wisdom. We see how intergenerational ties contribute to a feeling of continuity, purpose, and shared cultural identity. The age of silver becomes a witness to the richness of Nicoya's collective memory via rituals, storytelling, and community meetings.

The Peninsula of Life begs us to enjoy a life well-lived in the embrace of Nicoya's landscapes and customs, where the echoes of Pura Vida resound through the past.

We find inspiration in the peaceful coexistence of tradition, environment, and community as we immerse ourselves in the vivid tapestry of Nicoya's culture—a tribute to the lasting spirit that characterizes the quest for longevity in this enchanting Blue Zone enclave.

Chapter 6: Ikaria, Greece: The Island Where People Forget to Die - A Timeless Odyssey of Wisdom and Wellness

We set sail for the mysterious island of Ikaria as the sun sets below the horizon, throwing a golden light on the cerulean seas of the Aegean Sea—a refuge where the passage of time is measured not by ticking clocks but by the rhythm of a life well-lived.

In this part, we travel across Ikaria's rugged landscapes, sun-kissed vineyards, and centuries-old towns, digging into the mysteries of a Blue Zone where the residents seem to defy the very notion of death.

The Ikarian Landscape: A Timeless Beauty on Canvas

Ikaria spreads before us like a painting painted with Mediterranean hues—a scene where olive orchards extend over undulating hills, small settlements cling to hillside ledges, and the scent of wild herbs dances on the wind. We immerse ourselves in the natural beauty that serves as both the background and the basis of Ikarian well-being, reflecting on the islanders' healthy connection with their environment.

Earthly Nutrition: The Ikarian Diet as Culinary Alchemy

The fascinating alchemy of the island's diet— a symphony of fresh vegetables, beans, olive oil, and native herbs—is at the core of Ikarian longevity.

We explore busy marketplaces and traditional kitchens, learning about the culinary traditions that have nourished Ikarians for decades. The Mediterranean diet, known for its heart-healthy features, is more than simply a diet; it is a celebration of the riches that the land and sea supply, nurturing not just longevity but also a deep connection to the earth's bounty.

Timeless Traditions: Festivals, Music, and Life's Dance

Ikaria comes to life with an energy that transcends time and space. We dive into the island's colorful traditions, including festivals that resound with the sounds of old rhythms, music that speaks to the soul, and dances that seem to carry inhabitants through the past.

These ancient traditions provide witness to Ikaria's celebration of life, serving as a source of joy, community, and cultural continuity, all of which contribute to the island's general well-being.

Extended Families and Enduring Bonds in the Ikarian Social Fabric

The notion of family in Ikaria goes well beyond nuclear units, covering extended relatives and close-knit communities. We wind our way down winding streets where neighbors are more than just acquaintances—they are an essential part of one's existence. The chapter progresses as we investigate the community meetings, shared meals, and deep feelings of connectivity that contribute to the social fabric of Ikaria, generating not just a sense of belonging but also emotional resilience.

The Secrets of Longevity on the Island of Centenarians

As we go through the centuries-old settlements, each stone giving testimony to the passage of time, we come across Ikarians who seem to have discovered the key to resisting aging. We investigate the elements that contribute to Ikaria's unusual concentration of centenarians, which range from an active lifestyle and an antioxidant-rich diet to a focus on community and a calm way of life. The chapter examines the complex interaction of these elements, demonstrating a holistic approach to lifespan that is profoundly ingrained in Ikarian culture.

Ikarian Apothecaries of Nature: The Power of Herbal Medicine

Ikaria shows itself to be a natural pharmacy, with botanical treatments handed down through centuries. We go to the island's hills, where wild herbs such as sage, oregano, and marjoram thrive, adding flavor to Ikarian food as well as therapeutic virtues. The chapter progresses as we investigate the knowledge of Ikarian herbalists, pondering the relationship between ancient therapeutic methods and the island's broader devotion to holistic well-being.

Ikarian Ikigai and Spirituality: Finding Meaning in Simplicity

We discover a spirituality that is profoundly woven into the fabric of everyday life in the peaceful nooks of Ikaria's monasteries and churches.

In this episode, we look at the role of religion and contemplation in Ikarian Ikigai—the feeling of purpose and satisfaction that comes from simplicity, connection to nature, and living in tune with one's environment. Ikarians find meaning in the simplicity of their existence via rituals, prayer, and a great appreciation for life's intrinsic beauty.

Ikaria pulls us to explore the skill of forgetting to die in its timeless embrace, where the echoes of old traditions resound through the years. Ikaria reveals itself not merely as a destination, but as a timeless odyssey—an invitation to embrace a life rich in pleasure, community, and the endless possibilities of a well-lived existence—as we travel its landscapes, relish its cuisines, and immerse ourselves in its cultural tapestry.

Chapter 7:Lessons Learned and Practical Applications:Making Your Longevity Blueprint

We find ourselves at a crossroads of knowledge and action as we draw wisdom threads from the Blue Zones we've visited—the rugged hills of Sardinia, the tranquil shores of Okinawa, the vibrant communities of Loma Linda, the verdant landscapes of Nicoya, and the timeless beauty of Ikaria. This last chapter is a call to action, an opportunity to weave the lessons learned into the fabric of our own lives, not merely a meditation on the incredible tales of longevity.

Synthesizing Blue Zone Wisdom: The Longevity Tapestry

Before we get into the practical applications, let's take a look at the timeless wisdom weaved within the Blue Zone stories.
The common threads that connect these various societies indicate key principles for living a long and fulfilling life:

Plant-Based Nutrition: A largely plant-based diet rich in whole foods is the cornerstone of lifespan in Blue Zones.

Strong social relationships and a feeling of community both contribute greatly to overall well-being.

Purposeful Living: A feeling of purpose, whether via ikigai, religion, or cultural traditions, gives life depth and significance.

Regular Physical Activity: A healthy lifestyle that includes everyday, natural exercise benefits both physical and mental health.

Stress Reduction: Mindful techniques such as Sabbath observance or the calm Ikarian approach help to reduce the burden of stress.

Nature Connection: A respect for nature develops a balanced interaction with the world around us.

Making Your Longevity Blueprint: Practical Applications

Let us now go on the road of practical applications, equipped with these insights. Consider this chapter to be a call to action—a road map for incorporating Blue Zones ideas into your everyday life.

1. Adopt a Plant-Powered Plate:

Increase your intake of veggies, fruit, and whole-grain foods.
Experiment with Blue Zone-inspired plant-based cooking.
Reduce your meat intake and look at plant-based protein sources.

2. Make Social Connections:

Improve current relationships and make new ones in your neighborhood.
Face-to-face contact should take precedence over digital communication.
Participate in group activities, clubs, or local events to increase your feeling of belonging.

3. Identify Your Ikigai:

Consider your interests, abilities, and what gives you delight.

Find hobbies or interests that are in line with your beliefs and give you a feeling of purpose.

Incorporate Ikigai into your everyday life, whether via employment, hobbies, or community service.

4. Make regular physical activity a priority:

Discover interesting types of exercise that correspond to your interests.

Include natural exercise in your daily routine, such as walking or cycling.

Create a workout plan that incorporates both aerobic and strength-training workouts.

5. Mindfully Manage Stress:

Incorporate stress-relieving methods into your routine, such as meditation or deep breathing.

Set aside time for rest and self-care.
Develop a resilient mentality, seeing obstacles as chances for progress.

6. Get in touch with nature:

Spend time outside, whether at a park, a nature reserve, or your garden.
Mindfulness may be practiced in natural environments by appreciating the beauty around you.
Consider hiking, gardening, or birding to strengthen your connection to the environment.

7. Adopt Blue Zone Rituals:

Incorporate Blue Zone customs, such as group meals, storytelling, or traditional holidays, into your daily existence.

Create frequent opportunities for introspection, such as via prayer, meditation, or gratitude practices.
Accept the concept of a weekly day of relaxation, withdrawing from the stresses of everyday life.

Seek Professional Advice:

Consult with a healthcare practitioner, a dietitian, or a fitness expert to customize these concepts to your specific requirements. Regular check-ups and screenings aid in preventive health care.

Conclusion: A Lifetime Journey

As we complete our investigation of Blue Zones, keep in mind that the route to longevity is a constant, developing one. Accept the lessons learned, adapt them to your circumstances, and incorporate them into your daily routine. The tales of Sardinia, Okinawa, Loma Linda, Nicoya, and Ikaria are invitations to create your own story of life and well-being. May your path be filled with meaning, pleasure, and the eternal knowledge of a well-lived life.